Herbs For Health And Healing

**

Copyright © 2013 by Prem Chhatwani

ALL RIGHTS RESERVED

This book or any portion thereof may not be reproduced or used in any manner whatsoever without express written permission of the publisher except for the use of brief quotations in a book review.

Contact pjan86@gmail.com

Disclaimer: This book is not intended as a substitute for the medical advice of your personal medical doctor. The reader should consult a physician before considering any alternate therapies, including chelation, weight loss, cancer and diabetic alternate treatments requiring regular monitoring and diagnosis.

The author and publisher have made every effort to ensure that the information in this book was correct at press time. This book is a simplified version of various treatments and ideas including author's personal experiences and results. Reader may have different experiences and results and hence should be watchful when proceeding with these treatments and procedures.

The author and publisher do not assume and hereby disclaim any liability to any party for any loss, damage, or disruption caused by errors or omissions, whether such errors and omissions result from negligence, accident, or any other cause.

Table of Contents

1. World's longest serving physician and educator!

2. Nature's Premium Nutrient for Healthy Blood Sugar

3. Cinnamon and Honey

4. The Cure for All Cancers

5. Late Dr Johanna Budwig's Recipe to Fight Cancer

6. Hydrogen Peroxide and its common Uses

7. Cure For Cold / Flu and More!

8. Triphala - wonderful herb-blend of 3 fruits.

9. These 7 Foods will do the Weight-Loss Work for You.

10. Ashwagandha

11. Ginger

12. Turmeric

13. Banaba Extract

14. Garlic

15. Ginseng

16. Homemade recipe to unclog your arteries!

17. Lipoic Acid for your ailing kidneys

18. Final Reminder

1. World's longest serving physician, author and educator!

At the age of 97 years and 4 months, Shigeaki Hinohara is one of the world's longest-serving physicians and educators. Hinohara's magic touch is legendary

Since 1941 he has been healing patients at St. Luke's International Hospital in Tokyo and teaching at St. Luke's College of Nursing. After World War II, he envisioned a world-class hospital and college springing from the ruins of Tokyo; thanks to his pioneering spirit and business savvy, the doctor turned these institutions into the nation's top medical facility and nursing school.

Today he serves as chairman of the board of trustees at both organizations. Always willing to try new things, he has published around 150 books since his 75th birthday, including one "Living Long, Living Good", that has sold more than 1.2 million copies.

As the founder of the New Elderly Movement, Hinohara encourages others to live a long and happy life, a quest in which no role model is better than the doctor himself.

Here is the summary of his teachings.

1) Energy comes from feeling good, not from eating well or resting and sleeping a lot!

2) All people who live long regardless of nationality, race or gender share one thing in common: None are overweight.

3) Always plan ahead.... for EVERYTHING, however small the details be.

4) No need to ever retire, but if one must, should be a lot later than 65.

5) Share what you know.

6) When a doctor recommends you take a test or have some surgery, ask whether the doctor would suggest that for his or her spouse or children!

7) To stay healthy, always take the stairs and carry your own stuff.

8) Pain is mysterious, and having fun is the best way to forget it.

9) Don't be crazy about amassing material things.

10) Science alone can't cure or help people.

2) Nature's Premium Nutrient for Healthy Blood Sugar

It might seem hard to imagine that a few herbs can help you win the battle of blood sugar imbalances but it's TRUE! Let's examine each of these super nutrients individually.

Gymnema Sylvestre

For more than 2000 years, people in India have used the herb Gymnema sylvestre to help control blood sugar. In fact, the leaves of this climbing plant are prized by practitioners of Ayurvedic medicine, the holistic system of healing developed in India and practiced by the renowned doctor, Deepak Chopra. The herb is also called "gurmar," which literally means "destroyer of sugar" in Hindi. This name describes the way that chewing the leaves interferes with your ability to taste sweetness. Because this amazing herb decreases the sensation of sweetness in many foods, it may reduce your cravings for sugary snacks.

Dr. K. Baskaran published a study involving patients who took 400 mg of Gymnema sylvestre extract daily for 18 to 20 months along with their oral medications. This group showed a significant reduction in their fasting blood sugar levels.

Cinnamon:

Believe it or not your kitchen probably already contains a key ingredient to help you control unhealthy blood sugar levels. Recent scientific discoveries prove that a commonly used spice helps regulate blood sugar in ways previously unknown. Scientists at the Maryland-based Human Nutrition Research Center were studying the effects of common foods on blood sugar. Dr. Richard Anderson, lead scientist and chemist, noticed that when patients ate apple pie…their blood sugar levels actually IMPROVED!

Further investigation revealed it was the CINNAMON in the apple pie that helped their blood sugar levels. Researchers discovered that cinnamon actually increases your glucose metabolism. It contains a compound called Methyl Hydroxy Chalcone Polymer, or MHCP for short, that works with insulin to help process glucose. In fact, a laboratory test conducted by the U.S. Department of Agriculture (USDA) showed MHCP increased glucose metabolism by roughly 20 times.

Here is more on Cinnamon!

"CINNAMON TO LOWER BLOOD SUGAR & CHOLESTROL & TRIGLYCERIDES

Want to keep your blood sugar down to lower your odds of developing diabetes? Or if you are diabetic, would you like to lower blood glucose further without extra drugs?

Try eating more cinnamon or taking cinnamon capsules.
That's the advice of Richard Anderson, PhD researcher at the US Department of Agriculture.
"I know of no other natural ingredient that has the power cinnamon does in controlling blood sugar".
he says in a radio interview with Jean Carper.
In fact, Anderson said he takes cinnamon to control his own blood sugar and normally high cholesterol with astonishing success. His cholesterol plunged 60 points after he started getting about ¼ teaspoon of cinnamon twice a day, he says.

Anderson has reported similar results in a group of 60 people with type 2 diabetes in Diabetes Care, a journal of the American Diabetes Association. In those getting as little as 1 gram of cinnamon (1/4 tsp twice a day), blood sugar dropped 18 to 29%, triglycerides fell 23 to 30%, LDL bad cholesterol went down 7 to 27% and total cholesterol 12 to

26%. That's comparable to what you can expect from statin cholesterol -lowering drugs, he says. And cinnamon, unlike drugs, has no side effects.

What's also amazing, says Anderson, is that the benefits of cinnamon lasted for 20 days after subjects stopped taking it. Whereas the benefits of statin drugs vanish very quickly after you stop taking them, he says. You can sprinkle cinnamon on cereals, put it in juices, use it in desserts such as apple pie and make tea using a cinnamon stick. You can also buy it in capsules. One good brand, he says, is Cinnulin – a highly concentrated water extract of cinnamon. The product has been developed in cooperation with the USDA and Dr. Anderson".

Banaba Leaf Extract:

People living in the Philippines, South Asia, and India have used brewed banaba leaf tea to help regulate blood sugar. Medical scientists traditionally believe that banaba leaf's beneficial effects on blood sugar are due to its high concentration of Corosolic Acid, a natural compound extracted from its leaves. Corosolic Acid mimics insulin by moving sugar out of your bloodstream and into your cells.
Numerous scientific studies have proven Banaba

leaf's effectiveness. In one study, patients with blood sugar concerns took a supplement containing banaba leaf or a placebo three times a day for four weeks. The placebo group had no change, but the banaba leaf group achieved very good results for blood sugar balancing.

Banaba has been a time tested herbal remedy for kidney and bladder problems. Recent studies show that it is also good for diabetes and obesity. The people in Philippines have traditionally used the banaba leaf to make tea not only for diabetes, but for kidney and bladder ailments as well. Recent studies have shown, however that the entire herb is useful in lowering blood sugar levels. There are indications that Corosolic Acid may not be the only active ingredient in the Banaba. In a study published by Edison Biotechnology Institute in Athens, Ohio, it was concluded that all the parts of Banaba tree had a glucose lowering effect and that the herb could be used not only for diabetes but for obesity as well.

I would like to add two vegetables that have shown promise in reducing blood sugar levels in Diabetics and they are OKRA and Bitter Gourd or Karela as known in India.

OKRA (Abelmoschus esculentus) is a vegetable.

3) Cinnamon and Honey

Honey is the only food on the planet that will not spoil or rot. It will do what some call turning to sugar. In reality honey is always honey.. However, when left in a cool dark place for a long time it will do what I rather call "crystallizing". When this happens I loosen the lid, boil some water, and sit the honey container in the hot water, turn off the heat and let it liquefy. It is then as good as it ever was. Never boil honey or put it in a microwave. To do so will kill the enzymes in the honey.

Cinnamon and Honey Making News:

Bet the drug companies won't like this one getting around. Facts on Honey and Cinnamon: It is found that a mixture of honey and Cinnamon cures most diseases. Honey is produced in most of the countries of the world. Scientists of today also accept honey as a 'Ram Ban' (very effective) medicine for all kinds of diseases. Honey can be used without any side effects for any kind of diseases. Today's science says that even though honey is sweet, if taken in the right dosage as a medicine, it does not harm diabetic patients. Weekly World News, a magazine in Canada, in its issue dated 17 January, 1995 has given the following list of diseases that can be cured by honey and cinnamon as researched by western scientists:

HEART DISEASES:

Make a paste of honey and cinnamon powder, apply on bread, instead of jelly and jam, and eat it regularly for breakfast. It reduces the cholesterol in the arteries and saves the patient from heart attack. Also, those who have already had an attack, if they do this process daily, they are kept miles away from the next attack. Regular use of the above process relieves loss of breath and strengthens the heart beat. In America and Canada , various nursing homes have treated patients successfully and have found that as you age, the arteries and veins lose their flexibility and get clogged. Honey and cinnamon revitalize the arteries and veins.

ARTHRITIS:

Arthritis patients may take daily, morning and night, one cup of hot water with two spoons of honey and one small teaspoon of cinnamon powder. If taken regularly even chronic arthritis can be cured. In a recent research conducted at the Copenhagen University, it was found that when the doctors treated their patients with a mixture of one tablespoon Honey and half teaspoon Cinnamon powder before breakfast, they found that within a week, out of the 200 people so treated, practically 73 patients were totally relieved of pain, and within a month, mostly all the patients who could not walk or move around because of arthritis started walking without pain.

BLADDER INFECTIONS:

Take two tablespoons of cinnamon powder and one teaspoon of honey in a glass of lukewarm water and drink it. It destroys the germs in the bladder.

CHOLESTEROL:

Two tablespoons of honey and three teaspoons of Cinnamon Powder mixed in 16 ounces of tea water, given to a cholesterol patient, was found to reduce the level of cholesterol in the blood by 10 percent within two hours.
 As mentioned for arthritic patients, if taken three times a day, any chronic cholesterol is cured. According to information received in the said Journal, pure honey taken with food daily relieves complaints of cholesterol.

COLDS:

Those suffering from common or severe colds should take one tablespoon lukewarm honey with 1/4 spoon cinnamon powder daily for three days. This process will cure most chronic cough, cold, and clear the sinuses.

UPSET STOMACH:

Honey taken with cinnamon powder cures stomach ache and also clears stomach ulcers from the root.

GAS:

According to the studies done in India and Japan, it is revealed that if Honey is taken with cinnamon powder the stomach is relieved of gas.

IMMUNE SYSTEM:

Daily use of honey and cinnamon powder strengthens the immune system and protects the body from Bacterial and viral attacks. Scientists have found that honey has various vitamins and iron in large amounts. Constant use of Honey strengthens the white blood corpuscles to fight bacterial and viral diseases.

INDIGESTION:

Cinnamon powder sprinkled on two tablespoons of honey taken before food relieve acidity and digests the heaviest of meals.

INFLUENZA:

A scientist in Spain has proved that honey contains a natural ' Ingredient' which kills the influenza germs and saves the patient from flu.

LONGEVITY:

Tea made with honey and cinnamon powder, when taken regularly, arrests the ravages of old age. Take four spoons of honey, one spoon of cinnamon powder, and three cups of water and boil to make like tea. Drink 1/4 cup, three to four times a day. It keeps the skin fresh and soft and arrests old age. Life spans also increase and even a 100 year old, starts performing the chores of a 20-year-old.

PIMPLES:

Three tablespoons of honey and one teaspoon of cinnamon powder paste. Apply this paste on the pimples before sleeping and wash it next morning with warm water. If done daily for two weeks, it removes pimples from the root.

SKIN INFECTIONS:

Applying honey and cinnamon powder in equal parts on the affected parts cures eczema, ringworm and all types of skin infections.

WEIGHT LOSS:

Daily in the morning one half hour before breakfast on an empty stomach, and at night before sleeping, drink honey and cinnamon powder boiled in one cup of water. If taken regularly, it reduces the weight of even the most obese person. Also, drinking this mixture regularly does not allow the fat to accumulate in the body even though the person may eat a high calorie diet.

CANCER:

Recent research in Japan and Australia has revealed that advanced cancer of the stomach and bones have been cured successfully. Patients suffering from these kinds of cancer should daily take on tablespoon of honey with one teaspoon of cinnamon powder for one month three times a day.

FATIGUE:

Recent studies have shown that the sugar content of honey is more helpful rather than being detrimental to the strength of the body. Senior citizens, who take honey and cinnamon powder in equal parts, are more alert and flexible. Dr. Milton, who has done research, says that a half tablespoon of honey taken in a glass of water and sprinkled with cinnamon powder, taken daily after brushing and in the afternoon at about 3:00 P.M. when the vitality of the body starts to decrease, increases the vitality of the body within a week.

BAD BREATH:

People of South America , first thing in the morning, gargle with one teaspoon of honey and cinnamon powder mixed in hot water, so their breath stays fresh throughout the day.

HEARING LOSS:

Daily morning and night use of honey and cinnamon powder, taken in equal

parts restores hearing. I eat a toast
with real butter and cinnamon
sprinkled on it and then spread a bit of
honey over it.

4) The Cure For All Cancers

(Be advised this is a summary of Dr. Hulda Clark's 583 pages book.)

She passed away few years ago but was a legend in her own way.

Who is Dr. Hulda Clarke?

Hulda Regehr Clark began her studies in biology at the University of Saskatchewan, Canada, where she was awarded Bachelor of Arts, Magna Cum Laude, and the Master of Arts, with high honors. After two years of study at McGill University, she attended the university of Minnesota, studying biophysics and cell physiology. She received her Doctorate degree in physiology in 1958. In 1979 she left government funded research and began private consulting on a full time basis. Eleven years later she noticed clues as to the cause of cancer.

Before publishing her books on Cure For Cancers, Dr Clark set a goal to cure at least 100 cancer patients to test her theory. She passed that mark in December of 1992. The cure has stood the test of time. Her research has proved that all cancers are caused by a certain Parasite, regardless of the type of Cancer. The parasite is human **intestinal fluke**. If you kill this parasite, the cancer stops immediately.

Typically this parasite lives in human intestine causing no harm. May be causing only Crohn's disease, IBS and colitis. However if this parasite settles down in liver, it causes cancer! Further, this happens with people who have isopropyl alcohol (IPA) in their bodies.

All cancer patients (100%) have IPA (the solvent) and this intestinal fluke parasite in their liver.

What is intestinal fluke parasite:

The scientific name is " Fasciolopsis buski". Fluke means "flat". These are family of flatworms. The parasite has been known since 1925. The adult parasite stays stuck to our intestine. If in liver, causing cancer, or in uterus, causing endometriosis, or in thymus, causing Aids, or in kidney, causing Hodgkin's disease. In normal healthy people the parasite does not survive.

Flukes and Isopropyl Alcohol:

People who have isopropyl Alcohol in their bodies, their liver is not able to kill these parasites and they begin to multiply. From eggs to adult stage these parasites then eat and suck your body fluids. As soon as they are adults a growth factor called *orthophosphotyrosine* appears. These growth factors make cells divide. Now you have a CANCER!

Purge The Parasite, Cure the Cancer:

The good news is when this fluke, the parasite is terminated, in 24 hours all *orthophosphotyrosine* is gone! Your Malignancy is gone. Your Cancer can not come back. You have won the battle for your life.   Then all we have to do a cleaning and repair job.

So basically:

1. Kill the parasite and all its stages (Eggs and all)

2. Stop letting isopropyl Alcohol into your body

3. Flush out the metals, common toxins and bacteria from your body.

The Solution - The Herbal Parasite Remedies:

Just for your information our body is full of worms and all kinds of parasites. For example:

 * **Eczema is due to round worms**

* **Seizures are caused by a single roundworm called** *Ascaris*, **getting into your brain.**

* **Schizophrenia and depression are caused by parasites in the brain.**

* **Asthma is caused by** *Ascaris* **in the lungs**.

* **Diabetes is caused by the pancreatic fluke called** Eurytrema.

* **Migraines are caused by the thread worm,** Strongyloides.

* **Acne is caused by** Leishmania.

* **Much of heart disease is caused by dog heart worm**, Dirofilaria.

And the list goes on!

Getting rid of all these parasites is impossible with clinical medicines. In addition these medicines have side effects like nausea and vomiting.

Now the Good News!

There are just three Herbs **if taken together** will kill over 100 types of parasites. No side effects or interference with any drug that you are already on. They are nature's gift to us.

* Black Walnut Hulls from Black Walnut tree.

* Wormwood from Artemisia shrub.

* Common Cloves from the clove tree.

These three herbs must be taken together to kill adult parasites and the eggs which will develop into adults if not killed.

So here is what we need to start:

* One ounce (30 ml) of pale green Black Walnut Hull Tincture Extra Strength. This is enough for three weeks. 2 ounce bottle costs about $13.79.

* One bottle (about 100 capsules) of wormwood (each capsule with 200-300 mg of wormwood). 365 mg 100 caps cost about $13.99.

* One bottle of freshly ground cloves (500 mg, 100 caps cost $8.49).

In addition to these herbs, two additional items, **Ornithine** and **Arginine** will improve this recipe. Parasites produce a great deal of ammonia as their waste product and is set free in our bodies. It is toxic causing insomnia by night and anxiety by day.

By taking **Ornithine** at bedtime, one would sleep better. **Arginine** should be taken in the morning as it gives alertness and energy.

Ornithine 500mg , 100 caps cost about $14.29.

Arginine 500mg, 100 caps cost about 11.79

Parasite Killing Program.

1. Black Walnut Hull Tincture Extra Strength: (Source: New Action Products, Self health resource center. See at the end contact information)

Day 1: Take one drop and put it in a 1/2 cup of water and sip it on empty stomach before meals.

Day2. Take two drops same way

Day3. Take 3 drops same as above

Day4. Take 4 drops as above.

Day5. Take 5 drops.

Day6. Take 2 tsp. all together in 1/2 cup of water. Sip it slowly. Don't gulp it. Add sweetening or fruit sauce and get it down within 15 minutes. (If you are over 150 pounds use 2-1/2 tsp or if over 200 pounds take 3 tsp).

You can use lukewarm water to evaporate some of the alcohol in the tincture.

Then on, 2 tsp. once a week for a year.

Take 500mg of niacinamide(from Self Health Resource Center, Spectrum Chemical Co.) to counteract effect of alcohol in the tincture. If you feel slight nausea for few minutes, walk in the fresh air or simply rest.

Note for Extremely ill or terminally ill Cancer patients:

Take 2 tsp. of this dose every hour for 5 hours. Follow this the same day or next day with Mop up program. if this gets you out of the hospital bed, repeat this every other day for 2 more weeks, before settling for maintenance program once a week. Include wormwood and clove capsules 10 of each with each treatment.

2. Wormwood Capsules (200-300 mg)
(Available from Kroeger Herb Products, New Action Products, Self Health Resource Center)

Day1: Take 1 capsule before supper (with water)

Day2: Take 1 capsule before supper (with water)

Day3: Take 2 capsules before supper (with water)

Day4: Take 2 capsules before supper (with water)

Day 5 & 6: Take 3 caps before supper(with water)

Day 7 & 8: Take 4 caps before supper (with water)

Day 9 & 10: Take 5 caps before supper (with water)

Day 11 & 12: Take 6 caps before supper (with water)

Day 13 & 14: Take 7 caps before supper (with water)

Day 15 & 16: Take 7 caps before supper (with water)

Then on once a week 7 capsules forever.

3. CLOVES:

(Available at Self Health Resource Center, Starwest Botanicals, Inc., San Francisco Herb and Natural Food Co. -ask for fresh.)

Grind your own for freshness or purchase from recommended sources. Each capsule should be about 500mg.

Day1: Take 1 capsule 3 times a day, before meals.

Day2: Take 2 capsules, 3 times a day, before meals.

Day 3 - 10: Take 3 capsules 3 times a day, before meals.

Then on, take 7 capsules all at one time, once a week for ever.

Additional supplements:

Take Ornithine at bedtime and take Arginine in the morning and daytime. (Available at Self Health Resource Center, Spectrum Chemical, Seltzer Chemicals)

Resources:

Kroeger Herb Products, Boulder, CO

800-225-8787   www.kroegerherb.com

New Action Products, Orchard Park, NY

800-455-6459   www.newactionproducts.com

San Francisco Herb & Natural Food Co. Fremont, CA

510-770-1215   www.herbspicetea.com

Self Health Resource Center, San Diego, CA

800-873-1663 or 619-409-9500   www.shrc.net

Seltzer Chemicals, Inc. Near San Diego, CA

800-735-8137   www.seltzerchemicals.com

Spectrum Chemical Co. Gardena, CA

310-516-8000 or 800-791-3210
www.spectrumchemical.com

Starwest Botanicals, Rancho Cordova, CA

800-273-4372   www.starwest-botanicals.com

Dr Hulda Clark's book " The Cure for All Cancers" explains the above procedures and has over 100 case histories cured of cancer using this protocol, including bone cancer, breast cancer and many other cancers.. This is a must read book and is available at Amazon.com, or contact me for details.

Important Contacts: (Dr. Hulda Clark has passed away)

1) **Carmen Meyers**. Lives in Lemon Grove, CA near San Diego.

She is a trainer and experienced Syncrometer user since 1995. She worked under late Dr. Hulda Clark for years. I understand she still will test human Saliva sample for parasites , etc for a fee. Sample can be sent by mail. Contact her at 619-644-8635. Pacific Time zone. She has a website http://www.ctsoriginals.com/

She also Runs "New Century Press" in Chula Vista, CA (Near San Diego, CA) I always found it easy to call her there at 1-800-519-2465 or 619-476-7400. email contact: sales@newcenturypress.com

2) **Arthur Doerksen**, (Near Vancouver, B.C.)

Box 2094, Abbotsford, B.C. Canada V2T 3X8

He is an Engineer. He has perfected the Syncrometer and Zapper as per Dr. Hulda Clark's Protocol. He has a website http://www.bestzapper.com I talked, to him. He himself had a bout with cancer twice. Call him at 1-888-533-7007 (Pacific Time). Appears to be very helpful.

3) Now you can get several products here. http://www.drclark.com/

4) Also you can check this site.

https://www.budwigcenter.com/store/anti-parasite

I have no association with them, but you can ask them any questions, if you like.

 Summary: I think people with Cancer should try this approach as it will not interfere with their regular treatment. Also people with IBS, Diabetes, etc will also benefit. If I can be of additional help please contact me. I am only information provider and not a medical advisor. For any medical questions, please consult your doctor.

If you would like a FREE copy of DVD " Conversations with Dr. Clark" please send $4.00 for a copy and mailing charges. Will ship within USA . Once you get it you are welcome to make copies and distribute as I am doing it. If I can even just help save one precious life, yours or your loved ones, I will earn my wings!
Contact : Prem Chhatwani

Email: pjan86@gmail.com

Disclaimer: Please be advised information provided here does not replace traditional medical care. When in doubt, always consult your doctor before proceeding with any herbal or alternate therapies. You are responsible for your own action.

4) Late Dr Johanna Budwig's Recipe to Fight Cancer

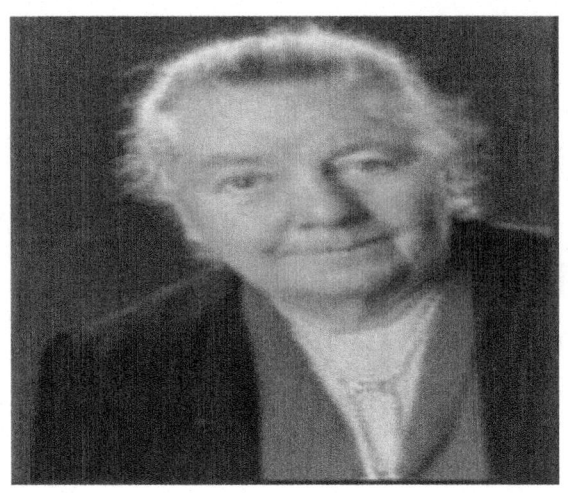

The Budwig Center teaches the **Budwig diet** founded by German biochemist **DR Johanna Budwig**. The Budwig Diet has been successfully helping people with Cancer, Arthritis, Asthma, Fibromyalgia, Diabetes, Blood Pressure, Multiple sclerosis, Heart Disease, Psoriasis, Eczema, Acne and other illnesses and conditions.

Here is the actual information from their site:

To make the Budwig Muesli, blend 2 Tablespoons of flaxseed oil (FO) with 4 Table spoons low-fat(less than 2%) Cottage Cheese (CC) with a hand-held immersion electric blender for up to a minute. If the mixture is too thick and/or the oil does not disappear you may need to add 2 or 3 Tablespoons of milk (goat milk would be the best option). Do not add water or juices when blending FO with CC. The mixture should be like rich whipped cream with no separated oil. Remember you must mix ONLY the FO and CC and nothing else at first. Always use organic food products when possible.

Next mix in by hand 1 teaspoon of honey (*raw non-pasteurized is recommended*)

(Optional) For variety you may add other ingredients such as sugar free apple sauce, cinnamon, vanilla, lemon juice, **chopped almonds**, hazelnuts, walnuts, cashews (no peanuts), pine kernels, rosehip-marrow. For people who find the

Budwig Muesli hard to take these added foods will make the mixture more palatable. Some of our patients have even added a pinch of Celtic sea salt and others put in a pinch of cayenne pepper for a change.

Note: I have very slightly modified the above procedure to make it easy. Take this sometime in the morning every day or any other time that works for you.

You will be surprised to start seeing benefits in 4-6 weeks. Do not discontinue.

Also since this is a food it should not interfere with your medication but if you are not sure please consult your doctor.

For additional research click on http://www.budwigcenter.com/anti-cancer-diet.php

Caution: Above information is not meant to replace the attention or advice of physicians or other health care professionals.

6. Hydrogen Peroxide and its common Uses

It is interesting to note that our digestive system produces H2O2. The baby gets a dose of H2O2 from colostrum from the first breast feeding. The falling raindrops contain H2O2.

There are several publications out there describing ever increasing uses of this wonderful product. Here are some you can try. Please use 3% H2O2 available from your local pharmacy. See my note at the end about food grade H2O2.

Caution: All these uses are not approved by FDA. However, you will be the sole judge and responsible for its use and results. Please do your own research and consult your medical advisor before using this product.

Cold and Flu symptoms:

At the first sign of cold insert 4 to 5 drops of 3% H2O2 in each ear. One ear at a time. Wait 3 minutes and let the liquid go in and create foaming effect. Some people feel ticklish! After 3 minutes, hold a tissue napkin on the ear and turn and wipe off the draining fluid. Repeat this now for the other ear. Repeat once if necessary after 8 hours or so.

Great for school kids as well in flu season. Just use fewer drops if necessary.

H2O2 Foot Soaks (Prepare as follows)

Water 20 parts
H2O2 3% 1 part
Salt One teaspoon (Epsom salt or Sea salt)
Time 20 minutes
After the soak scrub the feet to remove soft and white dead skin.

H2O2 Body Soaks: (Prepare as follows)

This is what I do as an adult (Follow your best judgment).
Fill the regular tub half with water with comfortable temperature and then pour into it 32 Fl Oz of 3% H2O2. You can start with 16 to 24 Fl Oz., initially if you like. Then simply move the water around to mix H2O2 and add some more water until it is enough to soak your body.

Make sure your neck, and face is above the water. Avoid contact with eyes directly.
Just soak for 20-30 minutes. Listen to some light music to relax.
After few treatments like this, next time add half to one cup of Epsom salt or Sea salt to water.
It will melt away your stress, help your aching joints and sore muscles, soften your skin and heal your minor cuts and wounds. In addition it will oxygenate your body.

H2O2 to Rescue in the Kitchen:

Prepare two spray bottles. One with 3% H2O2 and One with white vinegar (acetic acid). Sanitize everything in the kitchen, wood, metal and plastic surfaces including counter tops, cutting boards and any food preparation surfaces with these two sprays in any order you want. Both together have a tenfold power. Also spray on vegetables and meat before cooking.

Hydrogen Peroxide Therapies:

Among the alternate therapies, use of hydrogen peroxide (H2O2) to cure several ailments tops them all. There is wealth of information available on the worldwide web. Several books and articles are available on this subject as well.

However be advised that Hydrogen Peroxide therapies or Oxidation therapies as they are known are very controversial as for as main stream medical practitioners are concerned. There are few special doctors, MD's and N.D's who practice this. Some of them have been in trouble with their local medical state boards for doing this.

According to information I have gathered, hydrogen peroxide food grade has been used effectively to treat several diseases. It has been in use over past century. Doctors have infused dilute amounts into their patient's arteries, veins, noses, ears and mouths. It is a miracle food that provides oxygen to our sick cells in the body. Here are some quotes from medical doctors.

"Hydrogen peroxide is involved in all of life's vital processes.

It must be present for the immune system to function properly.

It is truly a wonder molecule."

William Campbell Douglass, M.D.

author of "Hydrogen Peroxide Medical Miracle"

"Hydrogen peroxide therapy can help achieve a multitude of therapeutic outcomes that would be unthinkable with a single drug or mainstream medical procedure. When levels of oxygen increase, the potential for disease decreases."

Nathaniel Altman, author of "The Oxygen Prescription"

Where to find a qualified doctor:

Here is the list of doctors worldwide who practice Oxygen therapies: Find the one you like and may be one near you. Be sure to check their practice and ask for testimonials, if you wish. Unfortunately most of them do not take medical insurance.

http://www.oxygenhealingtherapies.com/my_ozone_doctor.com.html

Here are some valuable comments I have collected for you:

GENERAL:

Hydrogen peroxide is NOT a "drug". Hydrogen peroxide is NOT a medicine. Hydrogen peroxide is a naturally-occurring substance that is made by Mother Nature and is also made by every cell in your body.

"It is a natural substance and therefore can't be patented. There is really nothing the drug companies can do about it except scare people into thinking that it is bad for them."

"When hydrogen peroxide is used as a therapeutic agent, it soon becomes obvious that it is useful in treating a wide variety of seemingly unrelated conditions."

CANCER:

"Hydrogen peroxide can act as an anti-cancer drug with two distinct advantages over conventional therapeutic agents: it produces minimal short and long term side effects and is relatively cheap and cost effective."

HEART DISEASE:

"Intra-arterial infusion of hydrogen peroxide has been noted to reverse the atherosclerotic process."

STROKE:

"I have had people coming into the office literally in the process of having a stroke. They are practically unconscious. We hook them up to the hydrogen peroxide, and an hour or two later, they walk out feeling fine."

THE FLU:

"The group treated with infusions of hydrogen peroxide missed a total of 5 days of work while the control group that received the conventional treatment missed 41 days of work."

EMPHYSEMA:

"It turns out that intravenous hydrogen peroxide can do something special, something that no other substance I know of can do. It can clean the lungs!"

IMMUNITY:

"Neutrophils have multiple systems available for killing ingested bacteria. Nearly all of these incorporate hydrogen peroxide, indicating its essential nature."

OXYGENATION:

"We can prove with blood samples that we can hyper oxygenate your blood stream better with hydrogen peroxide than by breathing oxygen. Better than by infusing ozone, better than by putting the patient into a hyperbaric oxygen chamber."

DENTAL:

"An expert advisory committee on antimicrobial agents found that hydrogen peroxide was the only substance that could safely and effectively be used for cleaning mouth injuries."

Hydrogen Peroxide (H2O2) As Mouthwash:

First thing in the morning when I start to brush I take about 1 oz. of 3% H2O2 in a cup and dip my brush into this for couple of seconds and brush my teeth with it. I repeat this couple of times each time dipping my electric tooth brush in 3% H2O2. I feel the foaming effect in my mouth.

Then I use my regular tooth paste to brush my teeth. To finish off, I add equal amount of water to remaining H2O2 and rinse and swish my mouth with it. I follow this same process before retiring at night.

Hydrogen peroxide as a mouthwash is lot cheaper than commercial mouthwashes on the market. In addition it will kill bacteria and viruses if used regularly. It is a great product to disinfect your gums and avoid gum diseases. I am a regular water- Pik user and I add 3 oz. cup of 3% H_2O_2 to the water Pik tank and then fill it up with water. Then simply jet spray between the teeth into the gums. I do this also as the last thing at night after brushing.

If you want to spend more money or simply do not like the taste of H_2O_2, there are commercial products containing H_2O_2 for you to buy and use. For example Colgate Peroxyl oral cleanser is one. It has 1.5% H_2O_2 and has a mint taste. However 8.0 FL Oz will cost you about $6.99. The product label description is as follows.

* Promotes the Healing of Oral Irritations

* Ready to Use

* Great Tasting Original Flavor

For the treatment of minor mouth and gum irritations.

Oxygenating action removes oral debris. This facilitates healing and alleviates discomfort.

Recommended by Dental Professionals for:

- Canker Sores
- Gum Irritations
- Denture & Mouth Sores
- Orthodontic Irritations
- Mouth Burns & Cheek Bites

Warning:

Do not use this product for more than 7 days unless directed by your dentist or physician. When using this product do not swallow. Reviews for this product are very positive except it is pricey!

My suggestion is to use 3% $H2O2$ and dilute it with equal amounts of water to make it 1.5% and use it as you would a commercial product. 8 Fl Oz would cost you about .25cents. The 3% commercial $H2O2$ comes in a dark brown bottle. You can make two bottles of 1.5% from this as long as you store it in a similar dark colored bottle. This way you can use it directly from the bottle, for the entire family. Encourage kids to rinse / swish their mouth after every meal or sweet desert and just before bed time. You will cut down your trips to your dentist and save money as well.

Hydrogen Peroxide Used in Many Grades:

Hydrogen Peroxide (H2O2) is available in many grades depending upon its use. Here is a quick review:

* 3% Hydrogen Peroxide available at your local drug store:

Used as disinfectant for cuts and wounds, as oral mouth wash and so on. Not for internal use. Contains stabilizers like phenol, acetanilide, Sodium Stanate and more.

* 6% Hydrogen Peroxide:

Used for coloring hair by beauty shops. Must have activator added to be used as bleach. Contains stabilizers, additives and impurities . Not for internal use.

* 30% Re-Agent Hydrogen Peroxide:

Used in medical research. Contains stabilizers, additives and impurities.

Not for internal use.

30-32% Electronic Grade Hydrogen Peroxide:

Used for cleaning electronic components and integrated chips before assembly. Contains stabilizers, additives and impurities. Not for internal use.

35% Food Grade Hydrogen Peroxide:

used for spraying inside of foil lined containers to store food.

contains stabilizers, additives and impurities.

90% Hydrogen Peroxide:

used by military as propulsion source in rocket fuel.

Note: Additives like Tin Stannate, Phosphate and Nitrate are added as stabilizers.

Tips to make your own 3% food grade Hydrogen Peroxide.

Buy 35% food grade H2O2.

Store it safely in your refrigerator with proper label to avoid accidents. Be careful when handling it as it will bleach your fingers.

For every 11 ounces of distilled water add 1 ounce of 35% H2O2 to make 3% H2O2. Use this as you would standard 3%. Store it in dark glass or heavy plastic bottle. I normally use the empty container of standard 3% bought from local pharmacy.

This food grade 3% H2O2 has less impurities. Some people even drink preparation made out of this. For example add one and half teaspoons of this 3% food grade to one gallon of distilled water. You can drink 1 Oz or more 3-4 times a day to oxygenate your body.

Caution: Please be advised we are not here to provide any medical advice. Do your own research and establish your own guidelines as with any alternate remedies. H2O2 is very effective sanitizer. It breaks down into water and oxygen and kills micro organisms by oxidation process.

Household uses:

Washing meat: Use salt and 3% H2O2 in chilled water for washing fish, poultry and meat to kill bacteria.

Washing Vegetables and salads: Use salt and 3% H2O2 to gallon of cold water. Wash all vegetables in this and then rinse with cold water to prolong freshness.

Laundry: Add 8 ounces of 3% H2O2 to your wash in place of bleaches.

Pets: For dogs and cats use 1 ounce of 3% H2O2 to a gallon of water for drinking and bath.

House and Garden Plants: Pour 1 ounce of 3% H2O2 in a quart of water. Spray and/or water plants with this mixture.

7) Cure For Cold / Flu and More!

Andrographis comes from India, Malaysia, Thailand, Indonesia, and Sri Lanka. This herb supercharges your immune system and helps flush out viral and bacterial infections. Here is just a sampling of what Andrographis can do.

Reduces Severity and Duration of Cold and Flu.

Historically, this herb has been used primarily as a treatment for cold and flu symptoms. Recent double blind human trials have proved that the use of Andrographis reduces not only the severity but also the duration of cold and flu.

Symptoms. Most people find that this herb relieves throat soreness, but researchers also noted that it improved other symptoms, including temperature, headache, muscle aches, cough, nasal symptoms, general malaise, and eye symptoms.

Helps Overcome Gum Disease

A new method of application for Andrographis is as a medication for periodontal disease and gingivitis. This condition is common among the elderly population, where individuals over 60 years old experience tooth loss due directly to periodontal disease. Research has proven that Andrographis is effective in inhibiting and killing the bacteria primarily responsible for periodontal disease, which prevents subsequent loss of teeth.

Beats Many Infections

Andrographis has been a staple to Ayurvedic medicine for thousands of years for its success in treating snakebites and overcoming malaria and dysentery. In traditional Chinese medicine, it is considered to be especially effective in clearing heat from the body and blood and is commonly used in treating heart conditions which include infection in the lungs, urinary tract, and throat (think strep throat).

Within the halls of Big Pharma, modern research has proven that Andrographis is beneficial for treating blood clots, stopping the spread of multiple types of cancer, and increasing the amount of immune enhancing white blood cells. Its active ingredients have been identified as Andrographolides. (Don't worry, chemists are still arguing over how to pronounce that correctly).

Thankfully, Big Pharma has failed miserably at designing a synthetic counterfeit of Adrographis. In its natural state, the wonder herb is always superior. Use it and say no to prescription drugs.

Making it Work for You

To make Andrographis work for you it must be taken in the right dose. One gram per 25 lbs body weight, split in three doses, should be consumed daily when cold symptoms arise or to prevent contagious infection. For instance, if you weigh 150 lbs then six grams daily is suitable - two grams three times per day. In health food stores, Andrographis is sold as a whole herb or as a 4-6% standardized extract of one of its active ingredients, Andrographolide. Anyone of these product variations is suitable.

Anything greater than a 6% extract should not be used, as it may be missing other naturally occurring ingredients that are vital for effectiveness.

Caution: Use alternate cures with care and do your own research. When in doubt consult your medical advisor. we are simply the information provider.

Andrographis comes from India, Malaysia, Thailand, Indonesia, and Sri Lanka. This herb supercharges your immune system and helps flush out viral and bacterial infections. Here is just a sampling of what Andrographis can do. Reduces Severity and Duration of Cold and Flu.

Historically, this herb has been used primarily as a treatment for cold and flu symptoms. Recent double blind human trials have proved that the use of Andrographis reduces not only the severity but also the duration of cold and flu

Symptoms. Most people find that this herb relieves throat soreness, but researchers also noted that it improved other symptoms, including temperature, headache, muscle aches, cough, nasal symptoms, general malaise, and eye symptoms.

Helps Overcome Gum Disease

A new method of application for Andrographis is as a medication for periodontal disease and gingivitis. This condition is common among the elderly population, where individuals over 60 years old experience tooth loss due directly to periodontal disease. Research has proven that Andrographis is effective in inhibiting and killing the bacteria primarily responsible for periodontal disease, which prevents subsequent loss of teeth.

8) Triphala wonderful herb-blend of 3 fruits

Triphala, an ancient herbal blend, is one of the most commonly used herbal remedies in the Ayurvedic system of healing. Ayurvedic medicine originated in ancient India. It has been developed over thousands of years, and is one of the oldest systems of healing. Thus Triphala is one of the longest-used herbal remedies in the world. Triphala, meaning "three fruits," is made from the fruits of three trees that grow throughout India and the Middle East, including Amalaki fruit (*Embelica officinalis*), Bibhitaki fruit (*Terminalia belerica*), and Haritaki fruit (*Terminalia chebula*). In preparing Triphala, these fruits are dried, ground into powder, and then blended together according to the precise directions of Ayurvedic tradition.

Amalaki fruit, also called Amla or Indian gooseberry, is renowned as one of the best rejuvenating herbs in Ayurvedic medicine. It contains more Vitamin C than almost any other fruit, consisting of nearly 3,000 mg of vitamin C per piece. It has been nicknamed the "nurse herb" in India, because of its widespread effectiveness against sickness and its cooling effects on the body.

Haritaki is also considered one of the most useful of Ayurvedic herbs, particularly for its rejuvenating, warming, and balancing effects. Combined with **Bibhitaki** fruit, another toning and warming herb, these three compounds are believed to have healing and balancing effects on all three of the principal body types or constitutions (termed Doshas) in Ayurvedic medicine. As a balanced formula, Triphala can be effectively used by most people and is prescribed for a variety of health conditions.

General Use:

Triphala is taken as a general health tonic, useful for all body types and a variety of conditions. It is commonly prescribed to tone and strengthen the digestive system, particularly in cases of weak digestion and constipation. It is a gentle laxative that can be used daily and is not habit-forming, and has no adverse effects on the intestinal flora (the microorganisms that aid digestion). It is said to improve the function of the stomach and intestines, and is also prescribed for cases of excess stomach acid. Triphala regulates and detoxifies the bowels, improves overall health by increasing the efficiency and absorption of digestion, and reduces gas. It has a balancing effect on the body's metabolism, and is prescribed to restore appetite. The herbal compound also helps the body to eliminate excess fat, by improving metabolism. Because of its gentle properties, Triphala is recommended as a digestive aid for the elderly and for those with sensitive stomach.

In addition to restoring the balance of the digestive tract, Triphala is used as a blood builder and purifier, and may increase red blood cell count and hemoglobin levels. Some healers prescribe it for diabetes, for its balancing effect on blood sugar levels. It also has anti-cholesterol and anti-mucus properties in the body. Triphala is believed to strengthen the kidneys and liver, and is prescribed for hepatitis sufferers.

Triphala is a source of vitamin C and is believed to improve the function of the immune system. The herbs in Triphala have anti-inflammatory properties. The remedy is prescribed for gout, a form of arthritis caused by excess uric acid in the body, and other inflammatory conditions. Triphala is said to have a calming and tonic effect on the nervous system, and is recommended for Alzheimer's disease and other degenerative disorders of the nervous system.

Another use for Triphala is to strengthen the eyes, particularly in cases of cataracts, glaucoma, and Conjunctivitis. It can be used as eyewash and may reduce soreness and redness in the eyes. Triphala can also be applied topically to the skin to speed the healing of bruises and sunburn.

Preparations:

Triphala is available as a powder, as tablets and in capsules form. For those who do not like very strong and bitter taste, tablets or capsules are recommended. Triphala can be taken daily. As a digestive tonic and laxative, it is best taken in the evening, about two hours after eating, and at least 30 minutes before bedtime. No food should be eaten for one and a half hours after ingestion.

Tablets and capsules can be swallowed, while the powder can be mixed thoroughly in a small amount of cold or warm water. The powder can also be simmered in water and consumed as a medicinal tea.

Individuals should start with small amounts of Triphala, a quarter-teaspoon of the powder or one tablet, gradually increasing the dosage until finding the optimal dosage. No more than one teaspoon of the powder or four to six tablets or capsules should be taken per day. The dosage should be reduced in cases of stomach upset or diarrhea.

As Triphala is not addictive, it can be taken over long periods of time. It is recommended that every ten weeks, users should stop taking the herbal compound for two to three weeks, to give the body a rest and to maintain the effectiveness of the remedy.

When used as eyewash, one teaspoon of Triphala powder can be added to one cup of hot water. The solids should be removed by straining through a dense cloth. The eyewash can be applied to the eyes three times per day. For topical application to the skin, the powder can be mixed with a small amount of water to make an easily applied paste.

Precautions:

Triphala is not recommended during pregnancy or nursing, and should not be used with cases of diarrhea and dysentery.

Side Effects:

The use of Triphala may increase intestinal gas at first, as a possible by-product of the cleansing and detoxification effects in the digestive tract. Loose stools or diarrhea may indicate too high a dosage, and the amount ingested should be reduced.

Interactions:

There are no known interactions between Triphala and standard Western prescription drugs as of 2004. **When in doubt, consult your medical advisor.**

9) These 6 foods will do the weight-loss work for you.

Over the course of the two-year study, the researchers found that boosting fiber by 8 grams for every 1,000 calories resulted in about 4 ½ pounds of weight loss.

1) A medium apple (3-inch diameter) contains 4 grams of fiber; a large apple (3¼-inch diameter) has 5 grams. Apples also offer a bit of vitamin C and potassium.

2) Green Beans : One cup boasts 4 grams of fiber, plus a healthy dose (30% daily value) of skin-helping vitamin C.

3) Sweet Potato: A medium-size baked sweet potato (2 inches wide, 5 inches long...a little larger than your computer mouse), skin included, offers 5 grams of fiber—for just 103 calories. It's also is a nutrition powerhouse: providing 438% daily value of eye-healthy vitamin A (eat these foods to help you see more clearly), 37% daily value of vitamin

C, plus some potassium, vitamin E, iron, magnesium and phytochemicals like beta carotene, lutein and zeaxanthin.

4) Raspberries: Raspberries are a great source of fiber—some of it soluble in the form of pectin, which helps lower cholesterol. One cup of raspberries has 8 grams of fiber. Raspberries are also an excellent source of vitamin C.

5) Strawberries: One cup of strawberries has a respectable 3 grams of fiber and more than a full day's recommended dose of vitamin C—an antioxidant that keeps skin healthy.

6) Chickpeas: Just ¾ cup of chickpeas has a whopping 8 grams of fiber! You also get a good amount of vitamin B6 and folate, both of which play a role in forming healthy new cells.

10) ASHWAGANDHA

Ashwagandha, a well known herb mostly cultivated in India and is easily available in USA. It is well known tonic and a stress reliever.

It is one of the most important Ayurvedic herb known.

In addition it is an excellent antioxidant and supports healthy immune system.

A 500mg dose can give you relaxing effect within few hours. It also has sex enhancing properties and improves endurance. There are no ill side effects. It can be taken over a long time. However it may not be a bad idea to take it for 2 weeks and then take a break for one week.

Other alternate is to take this 2 to 3 times a week.

It has pain suppressing qualities, and is effectively used to treat rheumatoid arthritis, osteoarthritis and gout.

It nourishes the brain and promotes calmness. It improves mental activity and concentration. It is often recommended for treating vertigo.

Improves stamina, slows aging process, has diuretic effect and is used in treating urinary infections. It is widely used to treat high blood pressure. It delivers strength to heart muscle improving heart functions. It is also used to treat respiratory infections and Asthma.

It is overall a great healing herb. Take it for all these benefits.

This herb is very affordable and is available widely at various health food stores or can be purchased over the internet.

Caution: Some people with thyroid problems should consult their doctor before starting on this herb. Also if you are taking several prescription drugs please seek advice from your health care provider.

11) GINGER

The Ginger or Ginger root is widely consumed in cooking recipes and very frequently used for its medicinal benefits around the world.

The Ginger root juice is very effective and Ginger root tea is frequently used with honey to treat cold, cough and abdominal pains or gas related symptoms. It is a blood thinner and has cholesterol lowering properties. It is also effective in treating Arthritis, diarrhea and nausea.

Ginger also has properties for relieving pain and reducing inflammation. Drink Ginger tea with your meal.

Over all safe by FDA, however it does interact with some medications like warfarin. Consult with your doctor if you are taking prescription drugs.

For Ginger Recipes search the web or explore this link

http://homecooking.about.com/library/archive/blspice10.htm

12) Turmeric

Turmeric is most famous as yellow curry powder. It is widely used in preparing Asian dishes. No kitchen should be without it.

Turmeric plant is from ginger family and mostly grown in South East Asia, including India. Commonly used in powder form in cooking.

Turmeric has many medicinal values and is used in Ayurvedic prescriptions.

U.S. National Institute of Health has currently more than 60 clinical trials underway for variety of medical disorders.

Some of these are for Alzheimer's disease, Cancer, Arthritis and anti-fungal properties.

Most common medicinal uses.

* Liver detoxifier

* As a pain and inflammation reliever.

* As a disinfectant for cuts and bruises.

* As a fat burner to reduce weight.

* Effective in reducing cholesterol, and in improving digestion.

*Antibacterial

*Treat depression

*Prevent heart disease

*Treat acne

*Treat rheumatoid arthritis

*Protect cardiovascular system

*Treat Alzheimer's disease

*Reduce tumor formation

*Regulate menstruation

*Treat eczema

*Treat stomach ulcers

*Treat gallstones

Apart from common use as a spice, which is the easier way to consume this yellow curry powder, here are few of my own uses I have personally used.

1) Add a dash of turmeric powder to warm milk and drink it then rest for reducing Allergies. This also helps in mild food poisoning.

2) Mix a small amount of the powder with body oil to make a paste and apply over cuts and wounds. It speeds healing.

3) I had a fall as a child and my arm was swollen. My Mom applied warm oil turmeric paste all over to reduce swelling.

Here is the link to interesting article on this curry powder and cancer.

http://in.reuters.com/article/2009/10/28/us-cancer-curry-idINTRE59R1E020091028

Here is another quote. "Curcumin (Turmeric) has for many years now been shown to reduce inflammation and to reduce oxygen toxicity or damage caused by free radicals in a number of experimental settings," said Dr. Jawahar Mehta, a cardiologist at the University of Arkansas for Medical Sciences in Little Rock.

"Taken in moderation or used in cooking, (curcumin) is quite useful," Mehta concluded.

13) BANABA EXTRACT

Banaba (not Banana) herb is cultivated widely in Philippines, India and Southeast Asia. It is frequently used for blood sugar control. The effect of Banaba extract is very much like insulin which helps transport glucose from the blood into body cells.

The active ingredient in Banaba Extract is Corosolic Acid known for its insulin like properties. If you are a type II diabetics consult your doctor for any interaction with your regular drug, before taking Banaba Extract capsules.

Several studies confirm that oral use of this herb helps reduce blood sugar levels in Type II diabetes. In addition it controls appetite, promoting weight loss as well.

The Banaba Extract is easily available from health food stores and normally comes with 1% or 2% Corosolic Acid in capsule form.

14) GARLIC

The famous Garlic comes from Onion family. It has been in use from ancient times and its use is often easily detected by its typical pungent flavor around kitchens and restaurants.

Though originated in Asia, it is widely used around the European nations and Africa as well.

It is commonly available as a bulb consisting of individual cloves.

While widely used as culinary ingredient, Garlic has many medicinal uses around the house.

Here are some claims worth making a note about.

1) Garlic is claimed to help reduce High Blood Pressure

2) It is also good for treating high Cholesterol

3) It is said to help regulate blood sugar

4) It is frequently used to combat cold and cough. Sip on to a hot cup of tea with few garlic cloves in it.

5) It has anti-fungal and antiseptic properties as well. It is that **allicin** in the garlic and several sulfur containing compounds in the garlic that are responsible for this.

It is interesting to note that some people believe that hanging a bulb of garlic outside the house or place of business wards off evil spirit. It must be that pungent smell!

Looking for Garlic recipes? Check out this site:

http://www.garlicrecipes.org/

15) GINSENG

Ginseng mostly comes from Korea and is also grown in North America, northern China and Eastern Siberia. Most popular variety in use is Panax Ginseng. There are other varieties including Siberian Ginseng.

Ginseng is available as dried roots. It can be orally taken as in a tea form or as in capsule form. It is important to use and buy authentic Panax Ginseng roots and not the dried leaves of this herb.

It is supposed to nourish the body, improve stamina, and improve sexual enhancement for men. Overall a good tonic, It is also beneficial for treating type II Diabetes.

American Panax Ginseng has similar properties and is easily available in health food stores. Ginseng is widely used in many herbal formulae to enhance the overall effect.

Ginseng Recipes:

1) Add Ginseng roots to your soups.

2) Ginseng Tea. Just add Ginseng tea packets available from your health food store to hot water and let it steep for 2-4 minutes. Add honey if you wish and enjoy.

3) For "Chicken Stew with Ginseng" and " Chocolate Peanut Butter Ginseng Cookies" visit this website.

http://www.wildgrown.com/index.php/Ginseng-Recipes.html

16) Homemade recipe will unclog your arteries!

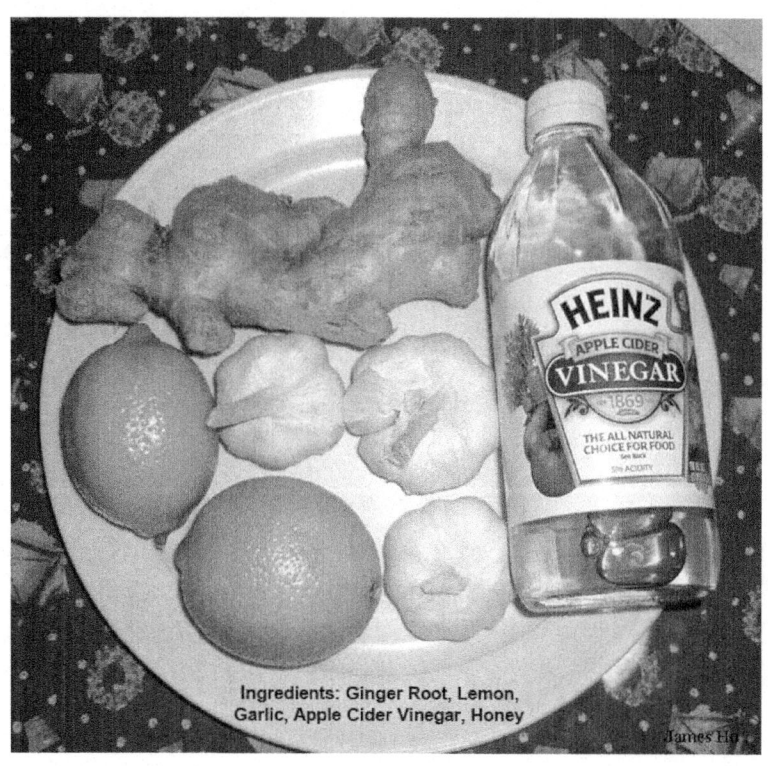

Ingredients: Ginger Root, Lemon, Garlic, Apple Cider Vinegar, Honey

Recipe for Opening Clogged Arteries.

1 cup Lemon juice, 1 cup Ginger juice, 1 cup Garlic juice
1 cup Apple cider vinegar

Mix all above and simmer in low heat for about 60 minutes or till solution reduces to 3 cups.

Remove solution to cool, then mix 3 Table Spoons of natural honey and store it in a jar.

Drink one tablespoon daily before breakfast. Your vein's blockage will open in most cases.
Enjoy your drink. Taste good too.

17) Lipoic Acid for your ailing kidneys

Kidney health know how: Your doctor will order a blood test that will measure "Creatinine" serum blood levels in addition to other tests. Healthy kidneys have creatinine levels between 0.6 to 1.2 mg/dl for males and 0.5 to 1.1 mg/dl for females. Young adults have higher readings compared to older people.

Higher creatinine levels indicate possible kidney issues that require medical attention. Some of the kidney issues may be due to dehydration, heart disease and bladder infections.

Unfortunately if and when kidneys fail and one cannot pass urine, the bladder is backed up and infection starts. You might feel tired, feel shortness of breath, and may be dehydrated. At this stage your doctor will put you on Dialysis, a treatment that will help clean your blood as it has impurities due to bladder back up. Several people I personally know about, mostly 60 and older have to take dialysis twice per week to stay functional.

So our goal would be to reduce Creatinine levels to normal range but at the same time look at the whole picture and seek out the causes of our kidney disease.

According to holistic approach, that is the purpose of this book, it will take another book like this to cover all that. However here are some tips to start with.

1) Meat and animal products have high creatinine, so switch to Vegetarian diet.

2) Cut down on intense physical workouts and exercise as these promote creatinine.

3) Avoid health supplements with Potassium and Vanadium.

4) According to some sources Alpha Lipoic acid supplement is very beneficial.

Here is more on Alpha Lipoic Acid:

Lipoic Acid is a unique vitamin supplement discovered in 1951. It is a Sulphur based compound. It has been used frequently to treat diabetes, kidney damage and Renal failure. It is water soluble as well as fat soluble hence has the ability to reach wherever body could use it.

Additional benefits:

1) Improves blood sugar control

2) Increases immune function

3) Helps eliminate heavy metals by binding with them in the liver

4) Improves energy

Lipoic Acid is available in three different forms.

1) R-Lipoic Acid: This is the most pure naturally occurring form. Best Buy.

Recommended dosage is 200mg /day to start and then increase up to 600mg/day.

2) Alpha Lipoic Acid: This is a blend 50-50 of natural and synthetic. Most commonly used form as it is also effective and affordable.

Recommended dosage: 400mg to start and may be work up to 600mg/day.

3) S-Lipoic Acid: This is the synthetic form. I would pass on this.

Note: Consult your health advisor as to which one is right for you and the correct dosage.

So this is a perfect nutrient for those suffering from kidney disease/failure caused by diabetes, cardiovascular issues, immune disorders and heavy metals.

In summary no matter what the reason Lipoic Acid is your natural best friend with amazing benefits for your ailing kidneys.

Foods that help kidneys: Broccoli, Spinach, Asparagus, Egg-Yolk, Brussels sprouts, brewer's yeast.

Herbs that Promote Kidney Health

Green tea - *Camellia sinensis* (Zingiberaceae) Native to the Orient, green tea has been consumed for thousands of years. The young, unfermented leaves of the green tea plant contain compounds known as *polyphenols* (plant antioxidants), which inhibit kidney stones and prevent cancers of the prostate, ovaries, liver, breast and colon. Green tea also helps the liver by reducing fatty deposits. Known to encourage improvement of the heart, circulatory system, brain, pancreas and liver, green tea also assists with weight loss by strengthening the metabolism via *thermogenesis* (an increase in body temperature that helps break down fat). Green tea also reduces cholesterol and is used as a heart tonic. Green tea is a stimulant (containing caffeine) and has anti-inflammatory, astringent and diuretic properties.

Java tea - *Orthosiphon aristatus* (Lamiaceae) or *Orthosiphon stamineus*
A shrub with lilac colored flowers, java tea is native

to Asia and Australia. The leaves of java tea (also known as *kidney tea* and *cat whisker plant*) are used medicinally. Java tea contains flavones (including *sinensetin*), glycoside (including *orthosiphonin*), volatile oil and large amounts of potassium. Java tea is listed in French, Indonesian, Dutch and Swiss pharmacopoeias as a remedy for kidney ailments including for conditions related to renal cleansing and function, and related disorders that include nephritis, cystitis, and urethritis.

Java Tea is used for kidney and bladder stones, liver and gallbladder problems and urinary tract infections. Java tea is also used as a way to reduce cholesterol and blood pressure. Java Tea is also taken for rheumatism and gout, although its effectiveness for these problems has not been verified.

Other names for Java tea include: Orthosiphon aristatus, Orthosiphon spicatus, Orthosiphon stamineus, Orthosiphonblaetter, Javatee, Indischer Nierentee, Feuilles de Barbiflore, and de Java.

18) Final Reminder

Always seek proper medical advice when following Alternate Therapies, if you have any doubts of the outcome.

Thank You.

Get All the Books in the Series

1) Pain Treatment with Magnets: Read Actual Case Histories.

[Kindle Edition]

http://tinyurl.com/n4ak2mj

2) How to Prevent and Reverse Heart Diseases- and Even Avoid   By-Pass [Kindle Edition]

http://tinyurl.com/k98q5b5

3) E D T A -This Four Letter Word May Save Your Life Using Chelation Therapy [Kindle Edition]

http://tinyurl.com/n7r7ge6

Printed in Dunstable, United Kingdom